I GOT IT! HERE'S WHAT TO DO ABOUT IT!

DIABETES

BY RORY CAROTHERS

TABLE OF CONTENTS

CHAPTER ONE: MY INTRODUCTION TO *"The Sugars"*

I can still remember the first time I heard someone mention "The Sugars." It was on a television show where an older Black woman referred to her illness as "the sugar." I didn't know then that "the sugar" was another term for diabetes—a silent killer lurking behind everyday symptoms. Hearing her talk about it left an impression on me, though. I thought diabetes was a condition that mostly affected older, overweight people, something that wasn't relevant to me or my lifestyle. That perception held up until I met a friend of mine in the Army who casually mentioned that they had diabetes.

This friend was in peak physical condition—fit, agile, and seemingly without any ailments. Seeing someone like them live with diabetes shook my assumptions and got me thinking that maybe this wasn't just a condition of the old or the unfit.

Physically, I've always been blessed. I was born with genetics that allowed me to stay muscular and athletic with minimal effort. My parents handed down this gift, so I didn't have to work too hard to maintain my physical fitness. I stayed active, ate well, and felt that my health was secure. But as I got older, even while serving in the Army, I started noticing subtle changes in my body. Instead of going to the doctor right away, I often brushed off these changes, coming up with my own explanations. There's a stereotype that men avoid doctors, but that wasn't me. I went to the doctor every chance I got—in the Army, we called it "sick call."

I'll never forget one particular visit. I was experiencing numbness in my limbs for the first time, and it alarmed me. But instead of an in-depth examination, I was handed a few Motrin and told to report back to duty. Over time, I started gaining weight, and my main health concern shifted to something else: sleep apnea.

But I didn't take it seriously. When you feel mostly healthy, it's easy to shrug off symptoms that seem manageable or unimportant.

At that point in my life, I didn't really understand depression, anxiety, or stress. I didn't know these could affect your physical body in profound ways. Yet over the years, I began to experience a range of issues: persistent headaches, dry or discolored patches on my skin, an insatiable thirst that left me feeling dehydrated all the time, and even more numbness in my limbs. I raised these concerns at different appointments, but each symptom seemed isolated—a headache here, some dry skin there, a little fatigue. I didn't make the connection that these symptoms could be linked.

It took time for me to piece it all together, but eventually,

I realized that these weren't just individual complaints —they were all clues pointing toward diabetes. I had experienced nearly all the classic symptoms without ever realizing that they were part of a larger issue.

CHAPTER TWO: MY WAKE-UP CALL

For years, doctors told me I was a "borderline diabetic," and somehow, I convinced myself that I would never actually get diabetes. I figured I was safe and that my body would always bounce back. After I left the military, though, my weight began to creep up steadily. No matter what I did, the scale refused to go down. I tried various diets, some exercise routines, and even supplements. But the truth was, I was in denial about the reality of my weight gain. I went from wearing large-sized shirts to a 2X, and then suddenly, I found myself buying 3X. Instead of facing the facts, I would look in the mirror and say, "Man, these 2X's are running small." It sounds almost funny now, but looking back, I see how I was doing some serious damage to my body by refusing to acknowledge the truth.

Even though I was in therapy, I wasn't managing my anxiety and depression as well as I could have. My mental health struggles were interwoven with my physical health issues, but I didn't realize how much these factors affected one another. Meanwhile, the symptoms of diabetes were manifesting in my daily life in ways I didn't recognize. There were warning signs that should have shown me how serious my situation was becoming.

One day, I was in a fast-food restaurant, and when my food was ready, I got up to grab it, but I felt a wave of dizziness and nearly blacked out. I brushed it off, thinking I just stood up too quickly. But in hindsight, I now know that dizzy spell was a symptom of my blood sugar levels being out of control. I had other symptoms, too— persistent numbness in my limbs, constant thirst, and unexplained fatigue. I visited the doctor repeatedly, had various tests done, but we couldn't pinpoint the cause. Looking back, it was all there; I just couldn't connect the dots.

Some of my friends had already lost loved ones to diabetes. Others had family members who faced life-altering consequences due to the disease, like amputations or blindness. Still, I remained in denial. My doctors would check my A1C levels, and when they told me it was around 6.5, they'd reassure me that I was "borderline" but "doing okay." And I took their reassurances at face value, convincing myself that as long as I wasn't officially diagnosed, I didn't have to worry too much.

Then, one winter, I got sick with a virus. Determined to avoid medicine, I tried every home remedy I could think of. Ginger ale became my go-to "medicine"—I drank it by the liter, thinking it would settle my stomach and get me back on my feet. Eventually, the virus passed, but I could tell something wasn't right. Even after recovering, I felt strange. Something was off, and for once, I couldn't ignore it.

Finally, I went to the doctor to address some of the lingering symptoms. After running tests, the results came back: my blood sugar had spiked to 254, and my A1C was sitting at a dangerous 10. According to the doctor, my blood sugar was high enough that I should have been in immediate danger of a stroke or insulin dependency. And yet, even with that alarming news, I still didn't fully grasp the seriousness of my situation. It took hearing how diabetes could impact every aspect of my life— including my sex life —for the gravity of my health crisis to truly sink in.

I realized then that if I didn't make drastic changes, the future I envisioned for myself might not be there. My path forward was clear: if I wanted to live a life free of medication and minimize my symptoms, I had to commit to a complete lifestyle shift. I needed to start eating right and exercising daily, no matter what. This wasn't just a temporary diet or a quick fix—it was a fundamental change to save my life.

That moment was my wake-up call, and from then on, I knew I had to face diabetes head-on. This battle wouldn't just be about my blood sugar levels; it would be a test of my determination to reclaim my health and well-being.

CHAPTER THREE: MY TURNING POINT

After receiving call after call from friends who'd seen recent photos of me, I finally had to face a hard truth. They were worried about my health, and it showed. They'd noticed my weight gain and weren't afraid to tell me that something seemed wrong. It struck me that people truly cared about my well-being. That realization was both humbling and eye-opening. It made me think: if others were this concerned, why wasn't I? And in that moment, I decided it was time to start caring about my health even more than they did. This would be a journey I took for myself, no one else.

Through mental health counseling, I began learning how to love myself unconditionally. I started to see self-care as an act of love rather than an obligation or chore. For so long, I had neglected my health, but therapy taught me that taking care of my body and mind was one of the deepest ways to honor myself. I stopped viewing exercise and healthy eating as things I *had* to do and began seeing them as choices I *wanted* to make because I valued my life and well-being. As a result, I started losing weight. But this time, it wasn't because of a strict diet or a quick-fix program. It was because I was finally understanding my own needs and making health a priority.

I want to issue a word of caution to you, dear reader: if you haven't learned how to cope with traumas from your past, or if you're still wrestling with depression, anxiety, or stress, these can derail you from your journey toward better health. I've been there. My own road to healthier eating and a better lifestyle was littered with fad diets, empty promises to myself, and the lure of quick fixes. I'd go all in for a few weeks, only to find myself sliding back into old habits. It wasn't until I truly began thinking about what my health meant to my family, friends, and children that I found the motivation to change. The thought of leaving my loved ones too soon or burdening them because of health complications was something I couldn't bear. That's when I began to take my health seriously.

I finally committed to taking the medication prescribed for my diabetes and to fully understanding how it worked. This wasn't an easy decision. Like many people, I'd resisted medication, thinking I could handle things on my own. But eventually, I realized that the medication was a tool to help me get my life back on track. I took the time to educate myself on how diabetes medication works, how it helps control blood sugar, and why it was essential for me at this stage. Once I embraced this part of the journey, I felt more empowered and in control.

Let me be honest with you: this journey isn't easy, and it isn't always fun. But what I can tell you is that it's absolutely possible. You can turn your life around if you're willing to take it one step at a time. I've put together some simple, straightforward exercises for those with busy schedules and those with a bit more time. I know firsthand that finding time for exercise can be tough, so I wanted to create routines that fit into anyone's life, no matter how hectic.

In addition, I've created a four-week meal plan designed to break the monotony of eating the same thing every day. I know how quickly "healthy eating" can become boring and discouraging if you're constantly eating bland meals. This meal plan includes a variety of flavors, textures, and nutrients, helping to keep things fresh and enjoyable.

This chapter marks my new beginning, a fresh start that I want to share with anyone who may be struggling as I once did. If you're ready to make a change, to love yourself in the deepest way possible, then this journey can be your new beginning, too. I hope my story and these tools can serve as a guide and a source of encouragement. Remember, it's never too late to start caring for yourself and embracing a life that's healthier, fuller, and genuinely rewarding.

CHAPTER FOUR: UNDERSTANDING DIABETES AND RECOGNIZING THE SYMPTOMS

As a veteran and as a man, I've come to realize that living with diabetes brings unique challenges and perspectives. For me, and for many others in similar positions, it can feel like more than just a diagnosis. It's a reminder to examine my lifestyle, habits, and health choices with a sharper focus. In order to take control of my condition, I needed to understand exactly what diabetes is and recognize the symptoms that come along with it. So, let's take a closer look at what diabetes truly means.

In addition, I've created a four-week meal plan designed to break the monotony of eating the same thing every day. I know how quickly "healthy eating" can become boring and discouraging if you're constantly eating bland meals. This meal plan includes a variety of flavors, textures, and nutrients, helping to keep things fresh and enjoyable.

This chapter marks my new beginning, a fresh start that I want to share with anyone who may be struggling as I once did. If you're ready to make a change, to love yourself in the deepest way possible, then this journey can be your new beginning, too. I hope my story and these tools can serve as a guide and a source of encouragement. Remember, it's never too late to start caring for yourself and embracing a life that's healthier, fuller, and genuinely rewarding.

CHAPTER FOUR: UNDERSTANDING DIABETES AND RECOGNIZING THE SYMPTOMS

As a veteran and as a man, I've come to realize that living with diabetes brings unique challenges and perspectives. For me, and for many others in similar positions, it can feel like more than just a diagnosis. It's a reminder to examine my lifestyle, habits, and health choices with a sharper focus. In order to take control of my condition, I needed to understand exactly what diabetes is and recognize the symptoms that come along with it. So, let's take a closer look at what diabetes truly means.

What is Diabetes?

Diabetes is a chronic medical condition that occurs when the body is unable to regulate blood sugar (glucose) levels effectively. Glucose is the primary source of energy for the body's cells, and insulin—a hormone produced by the pancreas—plays a key role in allowing glucose to enter those cells. When someone has diabetes, either their body doesn't produce enough insulin, or their cells don't respond to insulin properly. This leads to elevated levels of glucose in the bloodstream, which can have damaging effects over time.

There are two main types of diabetes:

1.   **Type 1 Diabetes**: This form of diabetes is an autoimmune condition where the body's immune system attacks the insulin- producing cells in the pancreas. As a result, the body produces little to no insulin. Type 1 diabetes often appears in childhood or early adulthood and requires regular insulin injections.

2.   **Type 2 Diabetes**: This is the most common form of diabetes and is typically related to lifestyle factors and genetics. In Type 2 diabetes, the body either resists the effects of insulin or doesn't produce enough to maintain normal glucose levels. This type is often linked to obesity, lack of physical activity, and poor dietary habits. Unlike Type 1, it usually develops in adults but is increasingly seen in younger individuals due to lifestyle changes.

Diabetes, particularly Type 2, has become a significant health issue worldwide, with millions affected. For veterans, like myself, the prevalence of diabetes is even higher due to a combination of factors, such as age, lifestyle changes post-service, and even exposure to certain chemicals like Agent Orange during combat. It's a condition that, if left unmanaged, can lead to serious health complications affecting nearly every part of the body.

Symptoms of Diabetes

Recognizing the symptoms of diabetes is crucial, as early detection can lead to better management and a lower risk of complications.
Many of these symptoms can seem minor or easy to dismiss, which is why I ignored them for so long. Here are some of the common symptoms associated with diabetes:

1.   **Frequent Urination**: High blood sugar levels cause your kidneys to work overtime to filter and absorb excess glucose. When they can't keep up, the excess glucose is excreted into your urine, dragging fluids from your tissues, which makes you urinate frequently.

2.   **Increased Thirst**: Because your body is losing fluids through frequent urination, you may feel excessively thirsty. It's a cycle that perpetuates itself—more urination leads to more thirst, and drinking more fluids leads to even more frequent urination.

3. **Unexplained Weight Loss**: Despite eating more, you may lose weight due to the body's inability to properly use glucose for energy. Instead, it starts burning muscle and fat for fuel, leading to weight loss.

4.   **Extreme Hunger**: Without enough insulin to move glucose into your cells, your muscles and organs become depleted of energy, triggering intense hunger.

5.   **Fatigue**: High blood sugar means your body can't use glucose efficiently, leaving you feeling constantly tired and drained, even with adequate rest.

6.   **Blurred Vision**: High glucose levels can pull fluid from the lenses of your eyes, affecting your ability to focus. If left untreated, diabetes can lead to more serious eye conditions and

even blindness.

7.   **Slow-Healing Wounds or Frequent Infections**: High blood sugar can impair blood flow and hinder your body's natural healing process, which can result in slow-healing sores, particularly on the feet and legs. This also makes you more susceptible to infections.

8.   **Numbness or Tingling in the Hands and Feet**: This is a symptom of nerve damage, known as neuropathy, that can occur due to prolonged high blood sugar levels. Left unmanaged, it can lead to severe pain or loss of sensation in these areas.

9.   **Dark Patches on the Skin**: Often found around the neck, armpits, or groin, these patches, known as acanthosis nigricans, are a common sign of insulin resistance.

For years, I experienced several of these symptoms, but I either didn't recognize them as warning signs or found a way to rationalize them. I brushed off my fatigue, attributing it to age or stress. I ignored my frequent thirst and frequent trips to the bathroom, thinking it was normal. Even the numbness in my hands and feet didn't set off alarms—it just became part of my routine.

Diabetes and Veterans: Unique Challenges

As a veteran, the journey with diabetes feels different from that of civilians. The statistics show that military veterans are at a higher risk of developing diabetes compared to the general population.
Nearly 25% of veterans in the VA healthcare system have diabetes, a rate that's nearly double the national average. This higher incidence can be attributed to several factors, including the stress of military service, changes in physical activity after discharge, and in some cases, exposure to chemicals or extreme conditions.

Veterans often face additional mental health challenges such as PTSD, depression, and anxiety, which can complicate diabetes management. For instance, the stress associated with mental health conditions can lead to unhealthy coping mechanisms, like overeating or neglecting exercise. As veterans transition from a regimented military lifestyle to civilian life, it's not uncommon to struggle with maintaining healthy habits, which can also contribute to higher diabetes rates.

Diabetes, a chronic condition characterized by elevated blood sugar levels, poses a significant health risk globally. Among military veteran men, the prevalence of diabetes is notably higher than in the general population. This chapter delves into the statistics surrounding diabetes in this demographic, exploring the underlying causes, associated health challenges, and the measures that can be taken to mitigate these risks.

Prevalence of Diabetes Among Military Veterans

Studies reveal that military veterans are disproportionately affected by diabetes compared to their civilian counterparts. According to the
U.S. Department of Veterans Affairs (VA), approximately **25%** of veterans in the VA healthcare system have diabetes, nearly double the prevalence in the general U.S. population. The incidence rate is even higher among older veterans and those who served in combat zones.

Factors Contributing to Higher Diabetes Rates
Several factors contribute to the elevated diabetes rates among military veteran men:

1.   **Age**: Many veterans accessing VA services are older, and age is a significant risk factor for diabetes.
2.   **Obesity**: Veterans may face challenges in maintaining a healthy weight post-service, with obesity being a major risk factor for type 2 diabetes.

Veterans often face additional mental health challenges such as PTSD, depression, and anxiety, which can complicate diabetes management. For instance, the stress associated with mental health conditions can lead to unhealthy coping mechanisms, like overeating or neglecting exercise. As veterans transition from a regimented military lifestyle to civilian life, it's not uncommon to struggle with maintaining healthy habits, which can also contribute to higher diabetes rates.

Diabetes, a chronic condition characterized by elevated blood sugar levels, poses a significant health risk globally. Among military veteran men, the prevalence of diabetes is notably higher than in the general population. This chapter delves into the statistics surrounding diabetes in this demographic, exploring the underlying causes, associated health challenges, and the measures that can be taken to mitigate these risks.

Prevalence of Diabetes Among Military Veterans

Studies reveal that military veterans are disproportionately affected by diabetes compared to their civilian counterparts. According to the
U.S. Department of Veterans Affairs (VA), approximately **25%** of veterans in the VA healthcare system have diabetes, nearly double the prevalence in the general U.S. population. The incidence rate is even higher among older veterans and those who served in combat zones.

Factors Contributing to Higher Diabetes Rates
Several factors contribute to the elevated diabetes rates among military veteran men:

1. **Age**: Many veterans accessing VA services are older, and age is a significant risk factor for diabetes.
2. **Obesity**: Veterans may face challenges in maintaining a healthy weight post-service, with obesity being a major risk factor for type 2 diabetes.

3.   **Physical Activity Levels**: Transitioning from active military service to civilian life often leads to a decrease in physical activity, contributing to weight gain and increased diabetes risk.

4.   **Mental Health Issues**: Conditions such as PTSD and depression, prevalent among veterans, are linked to unhealthy lifestyle choices and a higher risk of diabetes.

5.   **Exposure to Agent Orange**: Vietnam War veterans exposed to Agent Orange have an increased risk of developing diabetes, recognized as a service-connected condition by the VA.

Health Implications

Diabetes not only increases the risk of cardiovascular diseases, kidney disease, and neuropathy but also complicates existing health conditions common among veterans, such as hypertension and hyperlipidemia. The comorbidity of diabetes with other conditions requires a multifaceted approach to care.

Socioeconomic Impact

Diabetes among veterans poses a significant socioeconomic burden. The costs associated with managing diabetes —medications, frequent monitoring, and treatment of complications—are substantial.

Furthermore, diabetes can affect the quality of life, leading to disability and impacting veterans' ability to work, thus affecting their financial stability and overall well-being

VA Healthcare System and Diabetes Management

The VA has implemented various programs to manage and prevent diabetes among veterans:

1.   **Screening and Early Detection**: Regular screening for diabetes is a part of routine healthcare for veterans.
2.   **Educational Programs**: The VA provides education on healthy living, nutrition, and the importance of physical activity to prevent and manage diabetes.
3.   **Comprehensive Care**: Veterans diagnosed with diabetes receive comprehensive care, including access to endocrinologists, dietitians, and mental health professionals.
4.   **Telehealth Services**: The VA utilizes telehealth to provide remote monitoring and consultation, especially beneficial for veterans in rural areas.

CHAPTER FIVE: MY NEW UNDERSTANDING

Understanding diabetes and its symptoms has given me a new perspective. I no longer see these signs as isolated issues, but as interconnected pieces of a larger puzzle. For example, I now realize that my chronic fatigue wasn't just about getting older—it was a sign that my body was struggling to manage glucose. The numbness in my hands and feet wasn't something I could simply ignore; it was a symptom of nerve damage caused by prolonged high blood sugar. Recognizing this connection has been a wake-up call.

Living with diabetes means being vigilant and aware of how your body feels. It's about respecting your health enough to listen to the warning signs and taking proactive steps to manage the condition before it becomes overwhelming

Moving Forward

Now that I understand what diabetes is and the impact it has on my life, I'm prepared to take the steps necessary to manage it effectively. My journey involves not just controlling blood sugar, but also maintaining mental and emotional health. This knowledge has become my foundation for a healthier, more informed lifestyle, and I'm committed to doing what it takes to keep myself strong and healthy.

So, as we move forward together, let's remember diabetes isn't just about managing symptoms or taking medication. It's about taking control, educating ourselves, and making choices that honor our lives and our bodies. This understanding is my new starting point, and I hope it can be yours too.

I have included four weeks of meal plans. This is something that I am using as a guide. Please be aware of things you are allergic to and consult a doctor to determine what actions you need to take to address your weight and diabetes concerns. I am not a professional just a concerned citizen. Good luck on your journey let me know how you're doing on Instagram @soulfullexplorer. You got this!

CHAPTER SIX: THE MENTAL HEALTH BATTLE WITH DIABETES

Diabetes can impact mental health in profound and often unexpected ways. When I was first diagnosed as borderline diabetic, I didn't take it seriously. I didn't want to believe that something as straightforward as my blood sugar levels could threaten my life. But when I finally received a full diabetes diagnosis, reality hit me hard. For the first time, I faced an overwhelming concern about my own mortality. Am I going to live long enough to see my children grow? Will they have to face life without me? These questions stirred up a flood of fears that I had never faced before.

Alongside this fear, I felt a creeping sensation of depression. Instead of taking action, I found myself slipping into denial, avoiding the truth that demanded change. In my mind, I rationalized that all I had to do was "eat a little healthier," a vague plan with no real structure or intention.

This lack of planning created a dangerous cycle of avoidance and inaction. My mind was drained of the energy needed to motivate change, and I let the daily grind of life dictate my behavior rather than taking control. The shame of having diabetes kept me silent, and I felt isolated. I refused to share my diagnosis with friends or family and avoided conversations about health.

In this period, I was prescribed medication that felt harsh and intimidating, and I didn't like the aftereffects. I avoided taking it and stopped discussing my condition, even with those who could help. I clung to the belief that if I worked out, I could outrun diabetes—even if I wasn't fully committed to the dietary changes I needed. But without an integrated approach, my efforts fell short.

After a year of battling denial, it was a conversation with friends and doctors that finally nudged me toward a different path. I gathered the courage to see a nutritionist, something I had resisted. At that time, I was already working out with a trainer several times a week, but this was only one part of the puzzle. With the nutritionist's guidance, I began to realize how critical it was to align my mental and physical health. Facing my condition openly allowed me to accept the full reality of diabetes and understand that managing it required a consistent, well-rounded plan.

Battling diabetes means acknowledging the mental health component and understanding that depression, anxiety, and stress are common parts of the journey. I learned that seeking help is a sign of strength, not weakness. This journey is not just about blood sugar—it's about learning to care for myself holistically. Every time I start over, I gain new insights and strength. Today, with the right mix of medication, exercise, and nutrition, I'm finally seeing the progress I once thought impossible.

To anyone who's reading this, I urge you: Don't let shame silence you. Share your journey, seek help, and keep pushing forward. Diabetes doesn't have to define you, and with the right approach, it doesn't have to limit you either.

MEAL PLANS

Week 1
Day 1 - 7

- Breakfast: Rotate daily among:
  - Greek yogurt with berries and almonds
  - Scrambled eggs with spinach and whole-grain toast
  - Low-carb smoothie (spinach, cucumber, avocado, almond milk)
  - Oatmeal with walnuts and blueberries
  - Veggie omelet with bell peppers, onions, tomatoes
  - Overnight oats with chia seeds and cinnamon

- **Snack**: Options include apple slices with almond butter, celery with ranch, pistachios and peanuts, or cucumber with vinaigrette.

- **Lunch**: Choices like grilled chicken salad with mixed greens, a turkey wrap, or spinach salad with grilled chicken.

- **Dinner**: Options include grilled turkey breast with broccoli, chicken stir-fry with quinoa, baked chicken thighs with Brussels sprouts, and flank steak with brown rice.

Week 2
Day 8 - 14

- **Breakfast**: Choose from:
  - Scrambled eggs with spinach and bell peppers
  - Chia pudding with almond milk and berries
  - Veggie omelet with avocado slices
  - Smoothie (spinach, berries, almond butter)

- Boiled eggs with berries and nuts

- Snack: Options include strawberries with pecans, celery with ranch, a few squares of dark chocolate with raspberries, or cucumber with vinaigrette.

- Lunch: Options like lentil and vegetable soup, turkey lettuce wraps, and quinoa salad with grilled veggies.

- Dinner: Choices include stir-fried tofu with brown rice, baked chicken thighs with steamed green beans, stuffed bell peppers with ground turkey, and beef kebabs with vegetables.

Week 3
Day 15 - 21

- Breakfast: Repeat options from Week 1 to keep grocery shopping consistent.

- Snack: Similar to Week 1.

- Lunch: Choices like chicken and vegetable stir-fry, mixed greens with turkey slices, and black bean salad.

- Dinner: Rotate among grilled chicken thighs with cauliflower, baked tofu with kale, turkey meatballs with zucchini noodles, and grilled steak with Brussels sprouts.

Week 4
**Day 22 - 28

- Breakfast: Repeat options from Week 2 for variety and ease.

- Snack: Continue from Week 2 options.

- Lunch: Grilled chicken Caesar salad, turkey lettuce wraps, black bean and avocado salad, quinoa and roasted vegetable bowl.

- Dinner: Choices like grilled chicken with broccoli, tofu stir-fry with brown rice, turkey chili with bell peppers, and chicken fajita bowl.

Day 29 - 30 (to finish the month)

- Breakfast: Any favorite option from previous weeks.

ABOUT THE AUTHOR

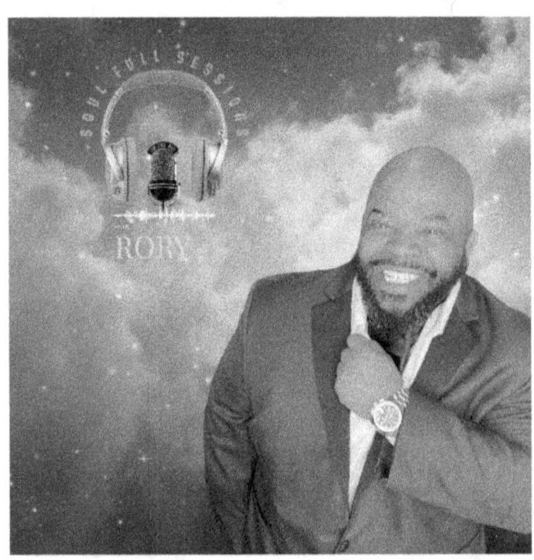

Rory Carothers, a Licensed Professional Counselor, brings a unique perspective shaped by years of personal experience and professional dedication. Known for his introspective approach, Rory delves into complex topics like mental health, resilience, and the intricate connections between physical and emotional well-being. His journey with managing diabetes has fueled his passion for guiding others toward healthier lifestyles and coping strategies. Through his work, Rory aims to empower individuals to embrace self-care, understand mental health's impact on the body, and navigate life's challenges with compassion and strength.

9 798346 607236